DR. ELIZABETH L. GEISLER

Change Your Diet For Optimal Mental Health

Contents

Why you need this book

You wake up each morning feeling a heavy fog lingering in your mind, clouding your thoughts and dimming your enthusiasm for the day ahead. Every task feels like a Herculean effort, and joy seems like a distant memory. Anxiety gnaws at your insides, and stress weighs heavily on your shoulders, making it difficult to find solace in even the simplest of pleasures. You long for clarity, for peace, for a sense of inner calm that seems perpetually out of reach.

But what if I told you there's another way? What if I told you that by making simple changes to your diet, you could transform your mental well-being and reclaim the vitality and resilience you thought were lost?

Welcome to the journey of transformation—a journey where the foods you choose to nourish your body become the building blocks of your mental resilience and vitality. In the pages of this book, you'll discover the profound connection between what you eat and how you feel, and you'll unlock the keys to unlocking your mind's full potential.

This isn't just another book about dieting; it's a manifesto for reclaiming your well-being and embracing a life of vitality, purpose, and fulfillment. It's a call to action—a reminder that you have the power to change your life by changing what's on your plate.

So, are you ready to embark on this transformative journey? Are you ready to unlock the secrets to optimal mental health and reclaim your joy, your clarity, and your zest for life? If so, then join me as we explore the transformative power of food and embark on a path to a brighter, healthier, and more vibrant future.

About the Author

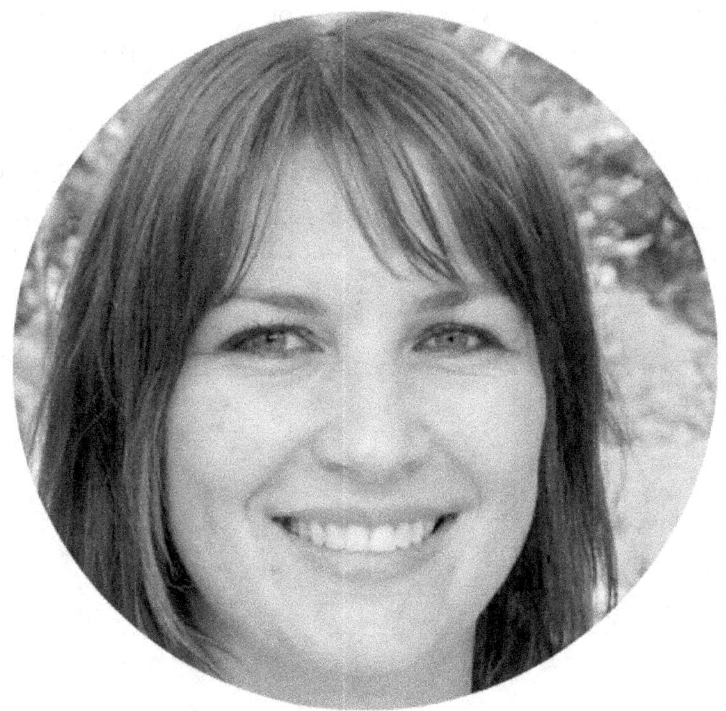

Dr. Elizabeth L. Geisler is a passionate advocate for holistic health and wellness. With a deep-rooted love for cooking and a keen interest in the intersection of nutrition and mental health,

she brings a unique perspective to the field. As a dedicated
mother of two, Dr. Geisler understands the importance of
nourishing both body and mind to foster a thriving family
dynamic.

Armed with a wealth of knowledge and experience in the realm
of nutritional psychiatry, Dr. Geisler is on a mission to empower individuals to harness the transformative power of food
for optimal mental well-being. Through her compassionate
approach and evidence-based insights, she guides readers on a
journey towards a healthier, happier life.

Dr. Elizabeth L. Geisler's dedication to merging culinary
creativity with mental health advocacy serves as an inspiration
to all those striving to achieve balance and vitality in their lives.

Understanding Mental Health

<u>What is mental Health?</u>

Mental health encompasses a person's emotional, psychological, and social well-being. It influences how individuals think, feel, and behave, as well as how they cope with stress, relate to others, and make choices. Mental health is not merely the absence of mental illness but also encompasses the presence of positive attributes such as resilience, self-esteem, and emotional intelligence.

Maintaining good mental health is essential for overall well-being and quality of life. It enables individuals to handle the ups and downs of life, form meaningful relationships, work productively, and contribute to their communities. Mental health is influenced by a combination of genetic, biological, environmental, and social factors, and it can fluctuate over time in response to various stressors and life events.

The Connection Between Diet and Mental Well-being

Throughout history, our understanding of the correlation between diet and mental health in the Western world has been incomplete. Observations by some individuals suggested a potential link between nutrition and overall health, both mental and physical. However, scientific validation was lacking.

In contemporary times, advancements in scientific research are shedding light on this relationship between food and mood. Increasingly, scientific evidence indicates a close connection between diet and mental well-being. Enhancing one's nutritional intake can directly impact symptoms of mental health disorders and contribute to overall mental wellness.

The exact prevalence of mental health conditions attributed to dietary factors remains uncertain. Nevertheless, depression stands out as one of the most widespread mental health disorders globally, with a significant portion of the population grappling with undiagnosed anxiety, depression, or both.

While a nutritious diet cannot serve as a cure-all for depression, making mindful dietary choices can ameliorate many symptoms associated with mental illness.

Nutrition Sustains Your Body

While it's common to primarily consider the physical effects of food, it's vital to recognize that your brain, immune system, neurological system, and endocrine system, among others, are all integral parts of your body. These interconnected systems play direct roles in aspects associated with mental health, such as stress regulation, mood modulation, and sleep patterns.

As human civilization has progressed, our bodies have adapted to derive nourishment from a diverse array of foods, including whole foods, raw foods, cooked foods, fermented foods, and minimally processed foods like whole wheat flour or natural peanut butter, as well as ultra-processed foods such as most freezer meals, fast food, cookies, and chips. However, the mere ability to derive sustenance from these foods does not guarantee optimal well-being. What you consume significantly impacts your overall health.

Your body relies on a complex blend of vitamins, minerals, antioxidants, fats, carbohydrates (for fiber and energy), water, and protein to operate efficiently. Some of these nutrients can be transformed into hormones and neurotransmitters that aid in bodily and mental regulation, while others facilitate cell repair and regeneration.

In the absence of these essential nutrients, the body prioritizes basic survival functions, often at the expense of mental well-being and energy levels. Therefore, the quality of your diet profoundly influences not only your physical health but also your mental and emotional vitality.

Understanding the Biological Basis of the Food-Mood Connection

Delving into the biological aspects of nutrition reveals how food significantly influences the body's stress management and mental health promotion.

Serotonin, known as the "feel-good" neurotransmitter or hormone, is crucial for regulating mood, sleep, appetite, and pain tolerance. Its production involves various steps in the gastrointestinal system, requiring specific nutrients like vitamin B1, copper, riboflavin, and calcium. Inadequate intake of these nutrients can lead to competition for resources within the body, potentially affecting certain systems.

The gut microbiome, composed of billions of beneficial bacteria, plays a vital role in producing essential vitamins such as B1 and neurotransmitters like serotonin. Communication between gut bacteria and the brain influences numerous bodily functions, including mental health. Recent studies show a connection between gut health and emotional well-being, with research indicating the impact of maternal gut microbiome diversity on the emotional health of offspring.

Additionally, inflammation, a natural immune response, can be worsened by certain foods like saturated fats, sugar, and unrecognized additives. Increased inflammation is linked to cognitive decline and dysfunction in brain regions like the hippocampus and amygdala, which regulate stress and the fight-or-flight response. Evidence suggests that chronic inflammation may contribute to mental health disorders such as depression and anxiety.

The nervous system, including the brain, spinal cord, and peripheral nerves, relies on various nutrients for optimal function. Omega-3 fatty acids, found in fatty fish and plant sources like walnuts and flax seeds, have anti-inflammatory properties and help manage neurodegenerative disorders such as Alzheimer's and Parkinson's diseases.

In essence, the complex relationship between nutrition and biological systems emphasizes the significant impact of diet on mental health. Acknowledging the importance of consuming nutrient-rich foods and maintaining a healthy gut microbiome is crucial for promoting mental well-being and resilience.

The Reciprocal Relationship Between Food and Mental Well-being

Our connection with food as humans is multifaceted. It serves as nourishment, pleasure, a social activity, and a source of comfort. Consequently, there exists a two-way link between diet and mental health. This means that mood can influence eating patterns, and conversely, eating habits can impact mood and psychological wellness.

Insufficient nutrition can intensify stress even in mildly stressful situations, leading to a tendency to opt for less nutritious foods for comfort or convenience to alleviate these feelings.

This unhealthy food choice further diminishes the capacity to cope with stress, fostering a harmful cycle of consuming foods that exacerbate feelings of anxiety.

A similar cycle can occur with depression, where low energy levels and a sense of depression prompt the consumption of soothing or effortless foods, often high in sugar and lacking in nutritional value. Post-consumption, one may feel even worse, perpetuating a cycle of deteriorating dietary and mental health.

A 2020 study published in The British Medical Journal conceptualized this relationship through three pillars and illustrated their inter relatedness:

1. High-quality diet – focusing on nutrition and reducing fast food consumption.
2. Physical health – maintaining good insulin sensitivity, a healthy cardiovascular system, and a healthy weight.
3. Mental health – experiencing improved mood, reduced stress, lower susceptibility to illness, and enhanced cognitive function.

Each of these factors influences the others, creating a feedback loop that can lead to the deterioration of mental and physical health as well as dietary habits. Enhancing mental well-being through nutrition entails breaking this negative cycle.

Research demonstrates the feasibility of this approach. A 2019 study revealed that increasing fruit and vegetable intake among individuals with mental health issues led to a reduction in symptoms.

Another study in 2022 investigated the impact of the Mediterranean diet on severe depression. Over a 12-month randomized controlled trial, the intervention group following the diet experienced a significant 20.6-point decrease in depression symptoms on the Beck Depression scale, compared to a 6.2-point decrease in the control group.

The Mediterranean diet emphasizes a variety of whole foods rich in fiber, vegetables, fruits, legumes, healthy fats, and fish, while minimizing or eliminating ultra-processed foods.

While the Mediterranean diet has gained traction, many diets worldwide share similar principles of prioritizing whole foods and minimizing ultra-processed foods.

The Emergence of Nutritional Psychiatry

Until recently, the relationship between diet and mental health was not widely understood in Western medicine. While ancient medicinal practices like Ayurveda in India and traditional Chinese medicine recognized the impact of food on both physical and mental well-being, Western medicine initially regarded this connection as vague and insignificant due to a lack of mechanistic understanding.

Psychiatric researchers primarily focused on developing medications and behavioral therapies to directly target brain chemistry and manage mental health conditions like depression and anxiety. However, a significant turning point occurred with a

1998 study revealing a strong international correlation between fish consumption and reduced depression rates. This prompted increased research interest in the link between diet and mental health.

Subsequent studies have further illuminated this connection, contributing to our understanding of how diet influences mental health and the prevention and management of mental health conditions.

Nutrition's Role in Mental Health Research

Numerous studies have demonstrated the association between nutrition and mental health disorders such as depression, anxiety, and ADHD.

For example, a 2014 randomized controlled trial showed that reducing inflammation through increased omega-3 intake could prevent certain types of depression. Additionally, a 1993 study found that lowering blood glucose levels in participants led to increased irritability and anxiety due to changes in counter-regulatory hormones like cortisol.

Poor dietary choices can contribute to insulin resistance, resulting in fluctuating glucose levels that may exacerbate anxiety symptoms in some individuals.

Furthermore, a 2018 study hypothesized that providing specific vitamins and minerals to children with ADHD could improve emotional regulation and reduce aggression. The results indicated significant improvements in the experimental group compared to the placebo group in areas such as attentiveness, aggression, and overall functioning.

Diet vs. Dieting

While prioritizing nutrition is crucial for mental health, it's essential to avoid extreme or restrictive dietary behaviors that could lead to adverse outcomes.

"Diet" refers to the overall pattern of food choices individuals make on a regular basis, emphasizing a balanced intake of nutrients for long-term health and well-being. Conversely, "dieting" often involves temporary and restrictive approaches aimed at achieving specific weight or health goals.

Opting for a healthy and balanced diet over short-term dieting approaches promotes sustained health and vitality.

Does Your Diet Impact Your Mental Health?

While further research is necessary to determine the most effective integration of nutrition and mental health treatment into an optimal diet, the abundance of well-designed studies overwhelmingly emphasizes the significance of nutrition.

Future investigations may unveil more tailored and personalized approaches for healthcare providers to systematically enhance their patients' mental health. However, individuals grappling with mental illness might discover that adhering to general nutritional guidelines can positively influence their mental well-being.

Enhancing mental health through nutrition necessitates a commitment to improving overall dietary habits. Currently, no pill, powder, or supplement can substitute for this. It's crucial to strive for obtaining most, if not all, nutrients from whole foods.

Anyone seeking to enhance their mental health via a more nutritious diet should always commence by consulting their physician.

Embarking on dietary changes is a significant decision that may involve societal, physical, emotional, and mental challenges. Sustaining these changes is easier if one has relative certainty about which foods or components may affect mental health positively or negatively. How can this certainty be achieved?

Commence a Food and Mood Diary

For a designated period, such as four weeks, meticulously record all food and beverages consumed. Additionally, record daily mood or the severity of mental health symptoms if formally diagnosed.

Upon completion of the period, analyze the data to identify potential patterns indicating a correlation between diet and mental well-being.

Systematically Introduce or Exclude One Component

The most effective approach is to select a substantial change. For instance, if one already avoids added sugar, completely eliminating it may not yield significant effects.

Individuals experiencing depression or anxiety who typically abstain from fatty fish might consider incorporating fish into their diet two to three times per week for four weeks. If fish consumption is not feasible due to dietary restrictions, plant-based alternatives can be chosen.

Subsequently, monitor symptoms daily. Do any changes in mood become apparent over time?

Introducing or eliminating one component serves as a gradual transition into a new dietary regimen. Depending on the outcomes during the trial period, one may choose to maintain the alterations, gradually incorporating additional dietary adjustments to further enhance nutrition and mental health.

Reduce Consumption of Fast Food and Ultra-Processed Foods

This adjustment may necessitate meticulous planning for individuals heavily reliant on ultra-processed foods. Advance planning is advisable to ensure access to nutritious alternatives during this period.

Some individuals might benefit from utilizing whole food-based meal kits for a week or seeking assistance from a supportive friend to learn how to prepare healthy, convenient meals.

Continuously monitor symptoms to assess any changes in mental well-being resulting from the absence or reduction of these foods in the diet.

Seek Professional Guidance

Considering substantial dietary modifications warrants consultation with a primary care physician (PCP) or a qualified dietitian. This ensures that informed and healthy choices are made throughout the process.

Fundamentals of Nutrition

Consuming food is vital for our existence, contributing to our social, physical, and mental welfare. However, numerous individuals overlook the importance of nutrition and lack a basic understanding of food's fundamental components. Food consists of calories derived from protein, carbohydrates, fats, or a blend of these components. Although water doesn't provide energy like calories, it is indispensable for the human body's functioning. Additionally, food provides essential vitamins and minerals in different proportions.

To comprehend the impact of dietary choices on our bodies, it's crucial to acquaint oneself with the fundamental principles of nutrition.

Macronutrients and Micronutrients

Dietitians and nutrition experts often categorize your diet into Macronutrients and Micronutrients.

Macronutrients encompass broad nutritional categories like carbohydrates, fats, and proteins, while micronutrients consist of individual vitamins and minerals such as calcium, zinc, and vitamin B-6.

You might be familiar with the term "counting macros," which involves a dietary strategy where individuals aim to consume a specific percentage of calories from each macronutrient group.

Continue reading to learn more about the research supporting this dietary method and how individuals incorporate it into their eating habits.

Micros versus Macros

The prefixes of these terms provide hints about their meanings. "Macro" is derived from the Greek word "makros," meaning large.

In nutrition, macros are typically quantified in grams, such as grams of fat or protein. Many diets focused on macros classify macronutrients into three categories:

Carbohydrates: present in foods like bread, pasta, and fruits, providing 4 calories per gram
    Fats: found in foods such as oils, nuts, and meats, providing 9 calories per gram
    Proteins: found in foods like eggs, fish, and tofu, providing 4 calories per gram
    It's worth noting that some diets consider alcohol as a separate macronutrient, offering 7 calories per gram. However,

due to its limited nutritional value compared to the other categories, some diets exclude it.

Micros, on the other hand, represent much smaller nutritional values. "Micro" originates from the Greek word "mikros," meaning small. Most Micronutrients are measured in milligrams or even micro grams.

The foods you consume contain numerous Micronutrients, particularly fruits and vegetables rich in vitamins and minerals. Examples of Micronutrients include:

- Calcium
- Folate
- Iron
- Vitamin B-6
- Vitamin B-12
- Vitamin C
- Vitamin E
- Zinc

While most macronutrient-rich foods also contain various micronutrients, a micronutrient-focused approach to dieting is uncommon because it would be challenging to measure and monitor.

How it Functions

Various approaches exist concerning daily macronutrient intake. For instance, the Dietary Guidelines for Americans offer the following recommendations concerning macronutrient distributions:

- 45 to 65 percent of daily calorie intake from carbohydrates
- 20 to 35 percent of daily calorie intake from fat
- 10 to 35 percent of daily calorie intake from protein

Individuals employing a macro-counting method as part of their dietary regimen typically start by determining their daily caloric requirements. Subsequently, they determine the proportion of calories from each macronutrient group based on their objectives.

For instance, individuals aiming to build muscle, such as bodybuilders, often consume higher proportions of protein, a crucial component for muscle growth. Conversely, those carefully monitoring blood sugar levels might opt for lower carbohydrate percentages to help stabilize their blood sugar levels.

The majority of scientific research on macronutrients involves analyzing an individual's diet and segmenting it into macronutrient components. This differs from instructing individuals to adhere to specific macronutrient quotas and observing whether they achieve weight loss or other objectives.

Consequently, from a scientific standpoint, it's challenging to determine the effectiveness or ease of adherence to a macro-based diet for the general population.

The Gut Brain Connection

The relationship between the gut and the brain is intricate and reciprocal. Communication flows in both directions between your digestive system and central nervous system, and the well-being or illness of one can influence the other. Essential components in this connection involve your enteric nervous system, your vagus nerve, and your gut microbiome.

Your brain and your gut engage in a continuous dialogue; if you've ever experienced a "gut feeling," you've sensed this interaction. This communication is evident when the anticipation of an exciting event induces "butterflies in your stomach," or when the prospect of something dreadful feels "gut-wrenching." Moreover, your gut sensations can impact your decision-making, often described as "going with your gut."

While your brain communicates with your entire body through nerves (your nervous system), it shares a unique bond with your gut. They converse about a wide array of topics, ranging from practical, physical matters to emotional ones. Surprisingly, more information flows between your brain and your gut than any other bodily system. Remarkably, there are more nerve cells in your gut than anywhere else in your body outside of your brain.

What is the significance of the gut-brain connection?

Over time, our brains and digestive systems have co-evolved to ensure our survival. The composition of our diets has varied significantly throughout history based on availability, making what we eat crucial for our overall health. Close communication between our brains and guts has been essential to ensure adequate nutrient intake and to signal when adjustments or caution are necessary.

This communication system includes the involvement of the emotional brain. Similar to how the emotional brain reacts to physical injuries to prevent future harm, it amplifies sensations in the gut, making them more noticeable. Heightened physical sensations can also lead to increased stress levels and emotional responses, creating a strong feedback loop between the brain and the gut.

What bodily functions does the gut-brain connection influence?

Research indicates that the interaction between the gut and brain can impact various aspects of our physiology and behavior, including:

- Appetite regulation and feelings of fullness.
- Preferences and cravings for certain foods.

- Sensitivities and intolerance to specific foods.
- Muscle movements involved in gut motility.
- Digestive processes.
- Metabolic functions.
- Mood regulation.
- Behavioral responses.
- Levels of stress experienced.
- Sensitivity to pain.
- Cognitive performance.
- Immune system function.

Which body systems contribute to the gut-brain connection?

The gut-brain axis, as healthcare providers term it, comprises a network of nerves linking the brain and gut, facilitating bidirectional communication. This intricate system involves not only the nervous system but also close interactions with the endocrine and immune systems.

The nervous system collaborates closely with the endocrine system, responsible for producing hormones that convey messages related to sensations such as hunger, satiety, and stress. Additionally, it interacts with the immune system to mount appropriate responses to gut-related injuries or illnesses.

Within this network, several key components play vital roles in the gut-brain connection:

Enteric Nervous System

Operating within the gastrointestinal tract, the enteric nervous system governs digestive functions, boasting over 500 million neurons, making it incredibly complex. Often dubbed the "second brain," it possesses a degree of autonomy from the central nervous system, enabling it to process and respond to local stimuli without relaying information to the brain.

Vagus Nerve

As one of the 12 cranial nerves, the vagus nerve serves as the primary conduit between the enteric nervous system and the brain. Transmitting sensory information from the gut to the brain and motor signals from the brain to the gut, it orchestrates various reflexes in response to changing conditions within the gut.

Gut Microbiome

Surprisingly, the gut microbiome, comprising bacteria residing in the gut, also contributes to the gut-brain connection. These microbes produce neurotransmitters and other chemicals that communicate with the brain, affecting mood and behavior. Moreover, alterations in the brain and gut can influence the gut microbiome by modifying its environment.

Recent research has unveiled the involvement of the gut microbiome in neurological, mental health, and functional gastrointestinal disorders, highlighting its significance in conditions like irritable bowel syndrome (IBS) and anxiety.

How Gut Health Influences Mental Health

The gut microbiota generates and interacts with various substances, including neurotransmitters such as serotonin and gamma-aminobutyric acid (GABA), which play essential roles in regulating mood and emotions. Serotonin, often referred to as the "happy hormone," is chiefly synthesized in the gut and influences mood, sleep, and appetite. Scharf points out that disturbances in the gut microbiota may hinder the production and transmission of these neurotransmitters, thereby contributing to mental health disorders. Research has uncovered elevated rates of depression and anxiety among individuals with gastrointestinal conditions like irritable bowel syndrome and ulcerative colitis.

Foods for Mental Clarity and Focus

Just as there isn't a miraculous solution to prevent cognitive decline, no single super food guarantees a sharp brain as you age. Nutritionists stress that adopting a healthy eating pattern is paramount, focusing on abundant intake of fruits, vegetables, legumes, and whole grains. Prioritize plant-based proteins and fish, and opt for healthy fats like olive oil or canola over saturated fats.

Studies indicate that the most beneficial brain foods are those that also promote heart and vascular health. These include:

Green, leafy vegetables:

Vegetables like kale, spinach, collards, and broccoli are abundant in brain-nourishing nutrients such as vitamin K, lutein, folate, and beta carotene. Evidence suggests that incorporating these plant-based foods into your diet may help decelerate cognitive decline.

Berries

Berries contain flavonoids, natural plant pigments responsible for their vibrant colors, which have been shown to enhance memory. A study conducted by researchers at Harvard's Brigham and Women's Hospital revealed that women who consumed two or more servings of strawberries and blueberries per week experienced a delay in memory decline of up to two-and-a-half years.

Tea and coffee:

The caffeine found in your daily cup of coffee or tea could provide more than just a temporary increase in concentration. A study published in The Journal of Nutrition in 2014 revealed that individuals with higher caffeine intake performed better on tests assessing mental function. Additionally, other research suggests that caffeine may aid in the consolidation of new memories. In a study conducted at Johns Hopkins University, participants were asked to study a series of images and then were given either a placebo or a 200-milligram caffeine tablet. The following day, a greater number of participants in the caffeine group were able to correctly identify the images.

Walnuts:

Nuts are renowned for their protein and healthy fat content, and one variety, in particular, may enhance memory. A study conducted by UCLA in 2015 found a correlation between increased walnut consumption and improved cognitive test performance. Walnuts are rich in alpha-linolenic acid (ALA), a type of omega-3 fatty acid. Diets abundant in ALA and other omega-3 fatty acids have been associated with reduced blood pressure and healthier arteries, benefiting both heart and brain health.

Recipes and Meal Ideas for Cognitive Enhancement

One-pan salmon with roast asparagus

- Preparation: 20 minutes
- Cooking time: 50 minutes
- Serves: 2

For a simple side dish to complement a spring roast, omit the salmon and prepare this recipe.

Ingredients:

- 400g new potatoes, halved if large
- 2 tablespoons olive oil
- 8 asparagus spears, trimmed and halved
- 2 handfuls cherry tomatoes
- 1 tablespoon balsamic vinegar
- 2 salmon fillets, approximately 140g/5oz each
- Handful of basil leaves

Method:

Step 1:

1. Preheat the oven to 220°C/fan 200°C/gas 7.
2. Place the potatoes and 1 tablespoon of olive oil in an ovenproof dish. Roast the potatoes for 20 minutes until they begin to brown. Add the asparagus to the potatoes and roast for an additional 15 minutes.

Step 2:

1. Add the cherry tomatoes and balsamic vinegar to the dish, and arrange the salmon fillets among the vegetables.
2. Drizzle the remaining olive oil over the salmon and vegetables. Return the dish to the oven for a final 10-15 minutes until the salmon is cooked.
3. Sprinkle the basil leaves over the dish and serve directly from the ovenproof dish.

Salmon & spinach with tartare cream

- Preparation time: 5 minutes
- Cooking time: 10 minutes
- Difficulty level: Easy
- Serves 2

Ever-versatile salmon is as popular on our shopping lists as chicken. Make the most of it with this impressive recipe.

Nutrition per serving:

- Calories: 321
- Fat: 20g
- Saturates: 5g
- Carbohydrates: 3g
- Sugars: 3g
- Fiber: 3g
- Protein: 32g
- Low in salt: 0.77g

Ingredients:

- 1 teaspoon sunflower or vegetable oil
- 2 skinless salmon fillets
- 250g bag spinach
- 2 tablespoons reduced-fat crème fraîche
- Juice of ½ lemon
- 1 teaspoon drained capers
- 2 tablespoons chopped flat-leaf parsley
- Lemon wedges, to serve

Method:

Step 1:

1. Heat the oil in a pan.

2. Season the salmon fillets on both sides.
3. Fry the salmon for 4 minutes on each side until golden and the flesh flakes easily.
4. . Transfer the salmon to a plate and let it rest while you cook the spinach.

Step 2:

1. . Place the spinach leaves in the hot pan.
2. . Season the spinach well, then cover and let it wilt for 1 minute, stirring occasionally.
3. . Spoon the wilted spinach onto plates and top with the salmon.
4. . Gently heat the crème fraîche in the pan with a squeeze of lemon juice, the capers, and parsley. Season to taste, being careful not to let it boil.
5. Spoon the sauce over the fish and serve with lemon wedges.

Basque-style salmon stew

- Preparation time: 10 minutes
- Cooking time: 25 minutes
- Difficulty level: Easy
- Serves 4

Heart-healthy salmon is the star of this straightforward one-pot dish, which contributes to your daily vegetable intake.

Nutrition per serving:

- Calories: 414
- Fat: 19g
- Saturates: 4g
- Carbohydrates: 29g
- Sugars: 11g
- Fiber: 5g
- Protein: 33g
- Low in salt: 0.33g

Ingredients:

- 1 tablespoon olive oil
- 3 mixed peppers, deseeded and sliced
- 1 large onion, thinly sliced
- 400g baby potatoes, unpeeled and halved
- 2 teaspoons smoked paprika
- 2 garlic cloves, sliced
- 2 teaspoons dried thyme
- 400g can parsley, optional

Method:

Step 1:

1. Heat the olive oil in a large pan.

2. Add the peppers, onion, and potatoes. Cook, stirring regularly, for 5-8 minutes until golden.
3. Add the smoked paprika, garlic, thyme, and chopped tomatoes. Bring to a boil, stir, cover, and simmer for 12 minutes. Add a splash of water if the sauce thickens too much.

Step 2:

1. Season the stew and place the salmon fillets on top, skin side down.
2. Cover with the lid and simmer for another 8 minutes until the salmon is cooked through.
3. Scatter with parsley, if desired, and serve.

Sardines & watercress on toast

- Preparation time: 5-10 minutes
- Difficulty level: Easy
- Serves 1

A nutritious and low-fat lunch option rich in omega-3 fatty acids. Feel free to substitute sardines with any other oily fish of your choice.

Nutrition per serving:

- Calories: 202
- Fat: 6g
- Saturates: 1g
- Carbohydrates: 23g
- Sugars: 0g
- Fiber: 3g
- Protein: 15g
- Low in salt: 0.85g

Ingredients:

- 1 slice of granary bread
- 1 garlic clove, halved
- 1 vine-ripened tomato, thinly sliced
- ½ can of Portuguese sardines in spring water, drained
- A handful of organic watercress or wild rocket
- A splash of balsamic vinegar

Method:

Step 1:

1. Lightly toast the bread.
2. . Rub the cut side of the garlic over the surface of the toast.
3. . Arrange the tomato slices on top and season if desired.

Step 2:

1. Break up the sardines with a fork and arrange them on top of the tomatoes.
2. Pile on the watercress and drizzle with balsamic vinegar.

Salsa spaghetti with sardines

- Preparation time: 15 mins
- Cooking time: 15 mins
- Difficulty level: Easy
- Serves 2

Canned fish from your pantry is a convenient way to incorporate omega-3 oils into your diet. Pair it with wholewheat pasta, tomatoes, olives, onions, and chili for a satisfying meal.

Nutrition per serving:

- Low in calories: 442
- Fat: 16g
- Saturates: 3g
- Carbohydrates: 43g
- Sugars: 10g
- Fiber: 7g
- Protein: 31g
- Salt: 1.7g

Ingredients:

- 100g wholewheat spaghetti
- 2 large ripe tomatoes, finely chopped
- 1 red onion, very finely chopped
- 15g pitted black Kalamata olives, quartered
- ½ tsp finely chopped red chili
- Zest and juice of ½ lemon, to taste
- 4 tbsp shredded basil or 1 tsp chopped fresh oregano
- 2 x 120g cans sardines in olive oil, drained (reserve oil if desired)

Method:

Step 1:

1. Boil the spaghetti according to the package instructions.
2. In a bowl, mix the chopped tomatoes, onion, olives, chili, lemon zest, and basil or oregano.
3. Heat the sardines either in the microwave or in a pan.

Step 2:

1. Drain the cooked pasta and return it to the pan.
2. Toss the pasta well with the tomato mixture.
3. Add the sardines in chunky pieces.
4. Season with lemon juice, pepper, and a little oil from the can, if desired.

Tomato and Spinach Chickpea Stew

- Preparation time: 10 mins
- Cooking time: 25 mins
- Difficulty level: Easy
- Serves 4

Create a cozy night in with this comforting dish, perfect for enjoying with some naan bread while lounging on the sofa.

Nutrition per serving:

- Calories: 145
- Fat: 6g
- Saturates: 0g
- Carbohydrates: 17g
- Sugars: 6g
- Fiber: 5g
- Protein: 7g
- Low in salt: 0.56g

Ingredients:

- 1 tbsp vegetable oil
- 1 red onion, sliced
- 2 garlic cloves, chopped
- ½ finger-length piece fresh root ginger, shredded
- 2 mild red chilies, thinly sliced
- ½ tsp turmeric

- ¾ tsp garam masala
- 1 tsp ground cumin
- 4 tomatoes, chopped
- 2 tsp tomato purée
- 400g can chickpeas, rinsed and drained
- 200g baby spinach leaves
- Rice or naan bread, to serve

Method:

Step 1:

1. Heat the vegetable oil in a wok and sauté the onion over low heat until softened.
2. Stir in the chopped garlic, shredded ginger, and sliced chilies. Cook for an additional 5 minutes until the onions are golden and the garlic is slightly toasted.

Step 2:

1. Add the turmeric, garam masala, and ground cumin to the wok. Stir over low heat for a few seconds.
2. Tip in the chopped tomatoes and tomato purée, then simmer for 5 minutes.

Step 3:

1. Add the chickpeas to the pan along with 300ml of water

(fill the can three-quarters full). Simmer for 10 minutes.
2. Stir in the baby spinach leaves until wilted.
3. Season with salt and pepper, then serve with rice or naan bread.

Mood-Enhancing Foods

We're familiar with the saying, "You are what you eat," but have you ever pondered that what you consume could influence your emotions as well?

Some foods are rich in vital vitamins, minerals, and compounds that can lift our mood. Enjoying mood-enhancing foods doesn't just promise mental health advantages; they can also enhance our physical well-being.

Let's explore 12 delightful foods that could add a little extra sunshine to your day and how you can incorporate them into your daily diet.

Dark Chocolate

Packed with flavonoids, dark chocolate has been associated with elevated serotonin levels, potentially aiding in relieving symptoms of depression.

Incorporate chunks into your breakfast oatmeal, stir it into your coffee, or simply indulge in a small piece as a post-dinner indulgence. Remember, moderation is important.

Bananas

These bright yellow fruits are rich in tryptophan, an amino acid that serves as a precursor to serotonin. Additionally, they contain vitamin B6, which assists in regulating mood.

Ideal for a quick and convenient snack, bananas can also be sliced over cereal, blended into smoothies, or incorporated into muffin recipes.

Berries

Strawberries, blueberries, and raspberries boast antioxidants that counteract oxidative stress, a factor associated with mood disorders.

These versatile fruits can enhance yogurt, enrich pancake batter, or provide a sweet addition to salads.

Oily Fish

Salmon, mackerel, and sardines

Salmon, mackerel, and sardines are packed with omega-3 fatty acids, renowned for their anti-inflammatory attributes and ability to alleviate depression.

Grilled salmon makes for a delightful dinner option. If you're craving something new, explore Japanese or Korean cuisine, where mackerel stars in dishes like grilled mackerel and spicy mackerel stew. For a quick yet flavorful snack, toss sardines into your salads or enjoy them on toast.

Nuts and Seeds

Walnuts, chia seeds, and flax seeds are excellent sources of omega-3 fatty acids. They're also versatile and can complement almost any dish when sprinkled on top.

Elevate your salads with walnuts or enjoy them as standalone snacks. You can also enrich your smoothies by incorporating chia seeds.

Oats

An ideal breakfast option, oats provide a gradual release of energy, helping to stabilize mood by avoiding sugar spikes and crashes.

Explore beyond traditional cooked oats. Try making overnight oats with fruits and nuts, crafting homemade granola or granola bars, or experimenting with savory oatmeal dishes featuring veggies.

Spinach

Packed with folate, a B vitamin essential for producing mood-regulating neurotransmitters like serotonin and dopamine, this leafy green is a nutritional powerhouse.

Incorporate a handful of spinach leaves into your homemade smoothies for a nutritious boost, or add them to your next omelette for a flavorful twist.

Avocado

Velvety and delightful, avocados are packed with B vitamins and monounsaturated fats, supporting neurotransmitter and brain health.

Spread it on toast, whip up some guacamole, or layer slices in salads and sandwiches. For a lusciously smooth treat, blend it into an avocado milkshake with milk, a hint of sweetener, and ice.

Green Tea

Packed with the amino acid L-theanine, green tea is believed to promote relaxation.

Green tea offers a mild caffeine kick to energize your mornings with clarity and alertness, balanced by the calming effects of L-theanine. This blend helps maintain mental focus without the typical jitteriness or agitation associated with caffeine alone.

Enjoy it hot to start your day or cold-brew for a revitalizing afternoon drink. It can also serve as a flavorful base for soups, such as thunder tea rice.

Beans

Packed with protein and fiber, beans play a crucial role in stabilizing blood sugar levels, warding off mood swings.

Utilize black beans for tasty taco fillings, while chickpeas can be roasted for a satisfyingly crunchy snack or blended into creamy hummus.

Poultry

Chicken and turkey are rich in tryptophan, promoting serotonin production and lifting mood.

Grill chicken breasts to add to salads or sandwiches, or opt for turkey as a lean choice in burgers or stir-fries.

Sweet Potatoes

Loaded with fiber and complex carbohydrates, sweet potatoes aid in stabilizing blood sugar levels and mood.

Whether roasted as wedges, mashed as a side dish, or stuffed with beans and veggies for a satisfying meal, sweet potatoes offer versatility and flavor.

Incorporating these mood-boosting foods into your diet not only adds variety but also has the potential to enhance your overall well-being. Remember, balance is essential. So, why not experiment with incorporating some of these mood-enhancing wonders into your next meal and observe how they positively affect your mood?

Nutritional Strategies for Managing Stress and Anxiety

As per the National Institute of Mental Health, anxiety disorders stand as the most prevalent mental health issue in the United States, affecting 40 million adults, which constitutes 18% of the population. Anxiety often coexists with depression, with approximately half of those experiencing depression also grappling with anxiety.

While specific therapies and medications can alleviate the symptoms of anxiety, only around one-third of individuals afflicted with this condition seek professional help. In my clinical practice, when discussing treatment options, I emphasize the significant role of diet in managing anxiety.

Alongside general healthy recommendations such as maintaining a balanced diet, staying adequately hydrated, and minimizing alcohol and caffeine intake, various dietary considerations can aid in alleviating anxiety. For instance, opting for complex carbohydrates, which are digested more slowly, helps regulate blood sugar levels, fostering a sense of calmness.

Opting for a diet abundant in whole grains, vegetables, and fruits proves to be a healthier choice compared to consuming excessive simple carbohydrates found in processed foods. Additionally, the timing of meals plays a crucial role. It's advisable not to skip meals, as doing so may lead to fluctuations in blood sugar levels, resulting in jitteriness that can exacerbate underlying anxiety.

The gut-brain axis holds significant importance, as approximately 95% of serotonin receptors are located in the gut lining. Ongoing research explores the potential of probiotics in treating both anxiety and depression.

Incorporating the following foods into your anti-anxiety diet can be beneficial:

- Magnesium-rich foods, such as leafy greens like spinach and Swiss chard, as well as legumes, nuts, seeds, and whole grains, may promote a sense of calmness, as low magnesium diets in mice have been associated with increased anxiety-related behaviors.
- Foods high in zinc, including oysters, cashews, liver, beef, and egg yolks, have been linked to reduced anxiety.
- Fatty fish like wild Alaskan salmon are rich in omega-3 fatty acids, which have been shown to potentially alleviate anxiety. A 2011 study on medical students was among the first to demonstrate the anxiety-reducing effects of omega-3s (in supplement form), following previous associations primarily with depression improvement.
- Asparagus, renowned for its health benefits, has gained recognition as a natural functional food and beverage ingredient with anti-anxiety properties, as approved by the Chinese government based on research findings.
- B vitamin-rich foods like avocado and almonds act as "feel-good" options, stimulating the production of neurotransmitters such as serotonin and dopamine. Incorporating these foods into your diet serves as a safe and simple initial approach to anxiety management.

Improving Mental Health with Dietary Changes

If you experience severe or prolonged anxiety symptoms lasting over two weeks, it's crucial to consult your doctor. Even if medication or therapy is recommended, it's worthwhile to inquire about the potential benefits of dietary adjustments. While nutritional psychiatry doesn't replace other treatments, the connection between food, mood, and anxiety is gaining increased recognition. With a growing body of evidence, further research is necessary to comprehensively comprehend the role of nutritional psychiatry, or as I like to refer to it, Psycho-Nutrition.

Foods for Sleep and Relaxantion

If the idea of sleep fills you with dread, consider examining your diet. Opting for the right foods before bedtime might significantly improve your sleep quality. Prioritizing good sleep can lower the risk of developing chronic illnesses, support brain health, and strengthen the immune system. Experts generally advise aiming for 7-8 hours of uninterrupted sleep each night, although many struggle to achieve this. Implementing dietary changes and consuming foods and beverages known to promote sleep can aid in enhancing sleep quality. Additionally, maintaining consistent meal times daily can be beneficial. Below are some recommended foods and drinks to consume before bed to optimize your sleep quality.

Almonds

Almonds are rich in various nutrients, making them a valuable addition to your diet. Regular consumption of almonds may decrease the risk of conditions like type 2 diabetes and heart disease, thanks to their healthy monounsaturated fats, fiber, and antioxidants.

Moreover, almonds could potentially enhance sleep quality. They contain vitamin B and magnesium, both of which can promote better sleep. Adequate magnesium intake, in particular, might improve sleep quality, especially for individuals with insomnia. Additionally, almonds, like other nuts, contain melatonin, a hormone that regulates your body's internal clock and signals the onset of sleep.

Although a study involving rats suggested that almond extract could increase sleep duration and depth, further research involving humans is necessary to confirm these findings thoroughly.

Turkey

Turkey is a flavorful and nutritious meat that is rich in protein, an essential component for maintaining strong muscles and controlling appetite. Additionally, it provides important nutrients such as riboflavin, phosphorus, and selenium.

Turkey contains tryptophan, an amino acid that stimulates the production of melatonin, a hormone that can induce drowsiness. This can potentially contribute to feelings of sleepiness.

The presence of protein in turkey may also play a role in promoting tiredness. Studies suggest that consuming moderate amounts of protein before bedtime is linked to better sleep quality, resulting in fewer disruptions during the night.

However, it is important to note that further research is needed to fully establish the potential impact of turkey on sleep improvement.

Chamomile Tea

Chamomile tea is a popular herbal beverage that has gained recognition for its potential health advantages.

One notable attribute of chamomile tea is its abundance of flavones, a type of antioxidants that can diminish inflammation, a common precursor to chronic ailments like cancer and heart disease. Moreover, chamomile tea possesses distinctive properties that might contribute to enhancing the quality of sleep.

Apigenin, an antioxidant present in chamomile tea, interacts with certain receptors in the brain, potentially inducing drowsiness and reducing instances of insomnia.

A study conducted in 2017 focused on elderly individuals, revealing that those who consumed 400 milligrams of chamomile capsules orally twice a day for four weeks experienced improved sleep compared to those who did not.

Nevertheless, additional up-to-date research specifically investigating the effects of chamomile tea on sleep may be necessary to glean more comprehensive insights.

Kiwi

Kiwi fruit is a highly nutritious and low-calorie option that can have several positive effects on your digestive health, inflammation reduction, and cholesterol levels. These benefits stem from the significant amounts of fiber and carotenoid antioxidants found in kiwis.

Furthermore, kiwis have been identified as a potentially beneficial pre-bedtime food. This is often attributed to the presence of serotonin, a neurotransmitter involved in regulating sleep cycles. Consuming a fruit-rich diet that includes kiwis may contribute to better sleep quality.

It has also been suggested that the sleep-promoting properties of kiwis may be linked to their anti-inflammatory antioxidants, such as vitamin C.

Nonetheless, further scientific research is necessary to fully understand the extent of kiwis' impact on sleep improvement.

Tart cherry

Tart cherry juice is a beverage that contains moderate levels of several essential nutrients, including magnesium, phosphorus, and potassium. It is also a plentiful source of antioxidants.

One notable attribute of tart cherry juice is its potential to induce sleepiness, primarily due to its elevated melatonin content. It has even been the subject of research investigating its effectiveness in alleviating insomnia. As a result, consuming tart cherry juice before bedtime may lead to improved sleep quality.

Nevertheless, further comprehensive research is required to substantiate the specific impact of tart cherry juice on sleep improvement and its role in preventing insomnia.

Fatty fish

Fatty fish, such as salmon, tuna, trout, and mackerel, are incredibly beneficial for our health. One of their standout features is their remarkable vitamin D content.

For instance, a 3-ounce (85-gram) serving of sockeye salmon provides 570 international units (IU) of vitamin D, which accounts for 71% of the recommended daily value (DV). Similarly, farmed rainbow trout offers 81% of the DV in a comparable serving.

Moreover, fatty fish are rich in omega-3 fatty acids, specifically eicosapentaenoic acid (EPA) and docosahexaenoic acid (DHA), which are renowned for their anti-inflammatory properties. When combined with the vitamin D present in fatty fish, these omega-3 fatty acids may contribute to safeguarding against heart disease and promoting brain health.

Walnuts

Walnuts are a popular variety of tree nuts that are highly nutritious and contain an abundance of healthy fats, including omega-3 fatty acids and linoleic acid.

Studies have been conducted on walnuts to explore their potential in reducing elevated levels of cholesterol, which is a significant risk factor for heart disease.

Moreover, some researchers suggest that consuming walnuts can enhance sleep quality, as they are among the best natural sources of melatonin, a hormone that regulates sleep.

Furthermore, a study conducted on mice has indicated that the fatty acid composition of walnuts may contribute to improved sleep. However, further research involving human subjects is necessary to substantiate the claims regarding the sleep-enhancing properties of walnuts.

Passionflower tea

Passionflower tea is an herbal infusion with a long history of traditional use in addressing various health conditions.

It serves as a valuable source of flavonoid antioxidants, which are recognized for their ability to reduce inflammation.

Furthermore, passionflower tea has been the subject of scientific research investigating its potential in alleviating symptoms associated with anxiety, depression, and other psychiatric disorders.

In particular, the findings of a small-scale study indicate that passionflower tea can enhance the production of gamma-aminobutyric acid (GABA), a brain chemical that inhibits the activity of stress-inducing neurotransmitters like glutamate.

The calming properties of passionflower tea may contribute to a sense of drowsiness, making it potentially beneficial to consume before bedtime.

White rice

White rice is a widely consumed grain that serves as a staple food in many cultures.

The main distinction between white rice and brown rice is that the former has undergone a process where the bran and germ are removed. This results in lower fiber content, reduced nutrient levels, and a decrease in antioxidants.

Nonetheless, white rice still contains a reasonable amount of certain vitamins and minerals.

White rice is primarily composed of carbohydrates. Its high carbohydrate content and lack of fiber contribute to its elevated glycemic index (GI).

Previous research, albeit older, has suggested that consuming foods with a high GI, such as white rice, at least one hour before bedtime, may contribute to improved sleep quality. However, it is important to note that these studies were conducted with professional athletes who may require higher carbohydrate intake compared to the average individual.

A review conducted in 2020, however, indicates that the evidence regarding the impact of high GI foods on sleep is inconclusive, highlighting the need for further research in this area.

Bedtime Snacks and Herbal Remedies for Relaxation

As the day winds down, nourishing bedtime snacks and soothing herbal remedies can promote relaxation and enhance the quality of sleep, contributing to overall well-being. Here are some options to consider:

Bedtime snacks:

1. Whole Grain Crackers with Nut Butter:

- Spread natural nut butter (such as almond, peanut, or cashew butter) on whole grain crackers.
- Optionally, drizzle honey or sprinkle cinnamon for added flavor.
- Serve and enjoy!

2. Greek Yogurt with Berries:

- Spoon Greek yogurt into a bowl.
- Top with fresh berries such as strawberries, blueberries, or raspberries.
- Optionally, add a sprinkle of granola or nuts for crunch.
- Serve chilled and enjoy!

3. Banana with Almond Butter:

- Peel a ripe banana and slice it into rounds.
- Spread almond butter on each banana slice.
- Optionally, sprinkle with chia seeds or cocoa nibs for extra texture.
- Serve as is or arrange on a plate for a simple and nutritious snack.

4. Oatmeal with Cinnamon:

- Cook oats according to package instructions (using water or milk of choice).
- Stir in a dash of cinnamon for flavor.
- Optionally, sweeten with honey or maple syrup if desired.
- Serve warm and enjoy a comforting bowl of oatmeal before bedtime.

5. Cottage Cheese with Pineapple:

- Scoop cottage cheese into a bowl.
- Top with chunks of fresh pineapple.
- Optionally, sprinkle with coconut flakes for added tropical flavor.
- Serve chilled and savor the creamy texture and sweet-savory combination.

6. Whole Grain Toast with Avocado:

- Toast whole grain bread slices until golden brown.
- Mash ripe avocado onto the toasted bread.
- Optionally, sprinkle with sea salt, red pepper flakes, or lemon juice for extra flavor.
- Serve immediately and relish the creamy goodness of avocado toast.

7. Warm Milk with Honey:

- Heat milk (dairy or plant-based) in a saucepan until warm but not boiling.
- Stir in a spoonful of honey until dissolved.
- Optionally, add a dash of vanilla extract or ground cinnamon for flavor.
- Pour into a mug and enjoy the soothing warmth of this classic bedtime beverage.

8. Cherry Tomato and Mozzarella Skewers:

- Thread cherry tomatoes and bite-sized mozzarella balls onto skewers.
- Optionally, drizzle with balsamic glaze or sprinkle with fresh basil leaves for extra flavor.
- Serve on a platter and enjoy a delightful combination of flavors.

9. Apple Slices with Peanut Butter:

- Slice apples into wedges or rounds.
- Spread peanut butter on each apple slice.
- Optionally, sprinkle with hemp seeds or chopped nuts for added crunch.
- Serve as a satisfying and nutritious snack.

10. Hummus with Veggie Sticks:

- Spoon hummus into a bowl.
- Cut raw vegetables such as carrots, cucumbers, bell peppers, and celery into sticks.
- Serve the hummus alongside the veggie sticks for a crunchy and satisfying bedtime snack.

These 10 bedtime snacks are delicious, nutritious, and easy to prepare, making them perfect for satisfying late-night cravings while supporting a restful night's sleep.

Herbal remedies:

1. Chamomile Tea:

- Place a chamomile tea bag or loose chamomile flowers in a mug.
- Pour hot water over the tea bag or flowers.
- Steep for 5-10 minutes, depending on desired strength.
- Optionally, add honey or lemon for sweetness.
- Sip and enjoy the soothing effects of chamomile before bedtime.

2. Lavender Pillow Spray:

- Fill a small spray bottle with distilled water.
- Add a few drops of lavender essential oil to the water.
- Shake well to combine.
- Spritz the lavender spray onto your pillow and bedding before bedtime.
- Allow the calming aroma of lavender to promote relaxation and improve sleep quality.

3. Valerian Root Tea:

- Place a valerian root tea bag or dried valerian root in a teapot or mug.
- Pour hot water over the tea bag or root.
- Steep for 10-15 minutes to extract the beneficial compounds.

- Strain the tea if using loose valerian root.
- Sip the warm valerian tea slowly before bedtime to induce relaxation and support restful sleep.

4. Passionflower Tea:

- Place a passionflower tea bag or dried passionflower in a cup.
- Add hot water to the cup.
- Allow the tea to steep for 10-15 minutes.
- Optionally, sweeten with honey or stevia if desired.
- Enjoy a cup of passionflower tea before bedtime to calm the mind and promote relaxation.

5. Lemon Balm Infusion:

- Place fresh or dried lemon balm leaves in a teapot or cup.
- Pour boiling water over the leaves.
- Steep for 5-10 minutes.
- Strain the infusion to remove the leaves.
- Optionally, add a slice of lemon or a teaspoon of honey for flavor.
- Sip the lemon balm infusion slowly before bedtime to soothe nerves and ease tension.

6. Peppermint Tea:

- Place a peppermint tea bag or dried peppermint leaves in a

cup.
- Pour hot water over the tea bag or leaves.
- Steep for 5-7 minutes.
- Strain the tea if using loose leaves.
- Optionally, sweeten with honey or agave syrup if desired.
- Enjoy a refreshing cup of peppermint tea before bedtime to relax the body and mind.

7. Linden Flower Tea:

- Place dried linden flowers in a teapot or cup.
- Add hot water to the teapot or cup.
- Steep for 10-15 minutes.
- Strain the tea to remove the flowers.
- Optionally, add a teaspoon of honey for sweetness.
- Savor the delicate flavor of linden flower tea before bedtime to induce calmness and promote sleep.

8. Catnip Tea:

- Place dried catnip leaves in a teapot or cup.
- Pour hot water over the leaves.
- Steep for 5-10 minutes.
- Strain the tea to remove the leaves.
- Optionally, add a teaspoon of honey for sweetness.
- Enjoy a cup of catnip tea before bedtime to relax the body and mind.

9. Skullcap Tincture:

- Fill a glass jar with dried skullcap leaves.
- Cover the leaves with high-proof alcohol, such as vodka or brandy.
- Seal the jar tightly and shake well.
- Allow the mixture to steep for 2-4 weeks, shaking the jar occasionally.
- Strain the tincture through a fine mesh strainer or cheese-cloth.
- Store the tincture in a dark glass bottle.
- Take 1-2 dropperfuls of skullcap tincture diluted in water before bedtime to promote relaxation and improve sleep quality.

10. California Poppy Tea:

- Place dried California poppy leaves and flowers in a teapot or cup.
- Pour hot water over the leaves and flowers.
- Steep for 10-15 minutes.
- Strain the tea to remove the plant material.
- Optionally, add a teaspoon of honey for sweetness.
- Enjoy a cup of California poppy tea before bedtime to ease tension and induce relaxation.

These herbal remedies can be easily prepared at home and enjoyed before bedtime to promote relaxation and support restful sleep. As always, it's important to consult with a healthcare professional before incorporating new herbs or supplements into your routine, especially if you have any underlying health conditions or are taking medications.

Lifestyle Factors for Optimal Mental Health

In essence, engaging in physical activity and exercise is crucial for individuals of all ages. Regardless of body type or BMI, children, adolescents, and adults alike benefit from regular physical activity to maintain good health. Recognizing the advantages of physical fitness and understanding the appropriate level of activity for your needs can contribute to overall well-being and enhance quality of life. Here are several benefits of consistent physical activity that underscore its significance in promoting health and vitality.

Cut Costs

As per the Centers for Disease Control and Prevention, chronic illnesses contribute to 7 out of 10 fatalities in the United States, with the treatment of these conditions comprising 86% of healthcare expenditures. While not all ailments are preventable, adopting a healthy lifestyle and minimizing risky behaviors can mitigate the likelihood of certain diseases like heart disease and diabetes.

Opting for healthy habits, such as incorporating regular physical activity into your routine, can diminish the risk of various health conditions and related complications, ultimately curtailing the need for costly medical interventions.

Prolong Your Life

Multiple studies indicate that maintaining a consistent regimen of physical activity can extend life expectancy and lower the likelihood of premature death. While there isn't a definitive equation equating hours of physical activity to additional years of life, research indicates that individuals who engage in regular physical activity generally experience better health outcomes and enjoy longer lifespans.

Minimize Injury Risks

Consistent exercise and physical activity bolster muscle strength, bone density, flexibility, and stability. This enhanced physical fitness not only reduces the likelihood of sustaining accidental injuries but also enhances resilience, particularly as one ages. For instance, improved muscle strength and balance diminish the chances of slips and falls, while increased bone strength mitigates the risk of fractures in the event of an accident.

Enhance Your Well-Being

A sedentary lifestyle and insufficient physical activity can adversely affect overall health. Physical inactivity is linked to heightened susceptibility to specific cancers, various chronic ailments, and mental health concerns. Conversely, regular exercise has been proven to uplift mood, enhance mental well-being, and offer a multitude of health advantages. Additionally, physical fitness enables individuals to engage in activities they may otherwise be unable to enjoy.

Maintain an Active Lifestyle

Prioritizing physical activity and maintaining good health enable individuals to participate in activities that demand a certain level of fitness. For instance, embarking on a challenging hike to reach a mountain peak offers a gratifying sense of achievement and breathtaking views. Unfortunately, fitness limitations can prevent some individuals from experiencing such joys.

Furthermore, even simple activities like strolling around the zoo with loved ones or playing on the playground with children can pose challenges for those who have neglected physical activity over time. By staying active, individuals make it easier to sustain activity levels as they age, enhancing their overall quality of life and enjoyment of diverse experiences.

Enhance Your Well-Being

Physical fitness offers a multitude of health benefits. Engaging in regular exercise and physical activity promotes the development of strong muscles and bones, enhances respiratory and cardiovascular health, and contributes to overall well-being. Moreover, maintaining an active lifestyle aids in weight management, lowers the risk of developing type 2 diabetes, heart disease, and certain cancers.

In essence, staying active is a pivotal component of sustaining good health and wellness. To support this endeavor, the Centers for Disease Control and Prevention (CDC) provides physical activity guidelines tailored to different age groups and life stages, including children, adults, older adults, and pregnant or postpartum women.

Encouraging your family to embrace physical activity and setting personal goals for daily or weekly exercise can foster a healthier lifestyle. Whether it's playing outdoor sports together, dedicating time for gym sessions, or adopting active hobbies such as hiking or cycling, there are countless ways to incorporate physical activity into your routine.

While National Physical Fitness and Sports Month serves as an opportune time to prioritize activity, the goal is to make exercise and physical activity a permanent fixture in your daily life. By doing so, you can reap the long-term benefits of improved health and vitality.

Gentle physical activities are less strenuous compared to

intense workouts or vigorous exercises. To gauge the intensity of physical activity, consider it moderate if you're able to sing while engaging in it. If you can talk but find it difficult to carry on a conversation, the activity is considered vigorous. Examples of light physical activities include walking, dancing, household chores, light weight training, yoga, and pilates. These serve as excellent alternatives to demanding exercises that may require more time and energy.

Here are 12 examples of light physical activities you can easily do at home. Studies indicate that substituting 30 minutes of sitting with moderate physical activities can lower the risk of premature death among individuals with low activity levels.

Consistently engaging in these activities also contributes to effective weight management. However, despite their moderate intensity, it's advisable to consult your doctor and undergo appropriate weight loss and fitness assessments to ensure the success of your fitness goals.

Here are some light physical activities you can easily do at home:

1. Household Chores:
   Engaging in household chores like cleaning, washing dishes, folding laundry, putting away groceries, dusting, ironing, and gardening may seem mundane, but they contribute to overall well-being. For example, vacuuming can burn 100-200 calories per hour, while doing laundry can help you burn 50-100 calories.

2. Couch Potato Workout:

This light physical activity can be done right from your couch. No equipment is needed. You can perform exercises like sitting-to-standing or try tricep dips by following these steps:

- Scooch forward on the edge of the couch.
- Place your hands backward on the edge of the couch.
- Lower your body.
- Lift yourself using your arms without your buttocks touching the floor.

3. Walking:

Walking is a simple yet effective everyday activity. Despite its commonality, its benefits for our bodies are often overlooked. According to the Anxiety and Depression Association of America, a ten-minute walk can be as beneficial as a 45-minute workout for relieving symptoms of anxiety. Additionally, walking stimulates creative thinking and cognitive functions, as highlighted by the American Psychological Association. It's cost-effective and suitable for individuals who may not have time for regular gym visits.

4. Plank:

The plank exercise may appear straightforward, but it targets multiple muscle groups and offers various difficulty levels. You can choose from different variations, such as planking with bent knees on the floor or attempting more challenging poses. An article in Physical Therapy Rehabilitation Science highlights the effectiveness of planks in strengthening core muscles, which play a crucial role in stabilizing the spinal column, aligning the body, and enhancing overall performance during movement.

5. Yoga:

Yoga is a recommended light physical activity that can be easily practiced at home due to its therapeutic benefits. It involves gentle stretching, balancing, and controlled breathing, requiring only a yoga mat or a soft cloth on the floor.

A study published in the NCBI journal suggests that yoga enhances muscular strength and body flexibility while improving respiratory and cardiovascular function. It also aids in addiction recovery and reduces stress, anxiety, depression, and chronic pain. Additionally, yoga promotes better sleep patterns and overall well-being and quality of life.

6. Dancing:

Dancing, beyond its role in entertainment, serves as a fun and enjoyable way to stay physically active, especially if traditional exercises are not preferred. Depending on intensity, dancing can burn 200 to 500 calories per hour on average.

Research indicates that dancing enhances flexibility, muscle strength and tone, endurance, balance, spatial awareness, and overall well-being. Specific dance movements, such as side-to-side motions and hip movements, contribute to bone strengthening, muscle toning, and improved posture.

7. Pilates:

Pilates can be practiced independently at home by following online tutorials or under the guidance of an instructor. All that's required is a yoga mat or towel.

Pilates is a holistic exercise method that aims to elongate, strengthen, and restore body balance through a blend of western and eastern body exercise techniques. Research suggests numerous health benefits associated with pilates, including improved posture, flexibility, circulation, balance, blood pressure, joint mobility, spinal health, and stress levels reduction.

8. Hula Hooping:

Hula hooping, particularly with weighted hoops, provides effective aerobic exercise, with the added resistance strengthening abdominal muscles. Consider choosing a hoop size that fits your body.

Studies have shown that practicing with weighted hula hoops can reduce abdominal fat and increase trunk muscle mass, particularly in overweight individuals.

These light physical activities, along with basic workout routines, offer moderate and highly tolerable exercises suitable for individuals looking to maintain a healthy lifestyle.

9. Squats and Lunges:

Squats and lunges are excellent choices for strengthening the lower body. These multi-joint exercises can elevate your heart rate and promote heavy breathing after just a few sets.

A study comparing balance and lower limb muscle activation during in-line and traditional lunge exercises found that split squats and lunges effectively increase hip and knee extensor muscle strength.

10. Side-Lying Hip Abduction:

Side-lying hip abduction is a simple yet effective exercise for strengthening the hip muscles without exerting excessive effort. It's best performed on a flat, stable surface.

- Lie on your side with both legs straight, one resting on the ground and the other on top.
- Lift and lower the top leg while maintaining proper body alignment, ensuring that the hips remain stable and the body stays straight.
- Repeat for the desired number of repetitions on each side.

11. Superman Exercise:

The superman exercise targets the lower back and posterior chain muscles, emphasizing proper form over speed.

- Lie on your stomach with arms and legs extended.
- Keep your neck in a neutral position to maintain spinal alignment.
- Engage your core and back muscles to lift your arms and legs off the ground as high as possible.
- Hold for a moment, then slowly lower back to the starting position.

12. 20-Minute Light Dumbbell Workout:

Research published in the Strength And Conditioning Research journal suggests that even lifting light weights can contribute to muscle mass gain.

For a quick yet effective workout targeting the biceps, triceps, and shoulders, try a 20-minute lightweight dumbbell routine. Perform each exercise for 15 to 20 reps, with a 15-second rest between sets, repeating for five rounds. This efficient workout allows you to maximize muscle engagement and achieve desired results without heavy lifting.

Here are two sample workouts you can incorporate into your routine:

Triceps Kickback:

1. Stand with feet hip-width apart, holding a dumbbell in each hand.
2. Hinge at the hips to achieve a flat back position, parallel to the ground.
3. Bend your arms to form a 90-degree angle, keeping your elbows close to your rib cage.
4. Extend your arms straight back without moving your shoulders, engaging your triceps.
5. Return to the starting position and repeat for the desired number of repetitions.

Uppercut Pulse:

1. Stand with feet hip-width apart.
2. Lift your arms to shoulder height, bending them at 90-degree angles with palms facing each other.
3. Pulse your arms up and down, alternating between bringing your hands above and below your head.

It's crucial to prioritize your health, especially when life gets busy. Neglecting physical activity increases the risk of various health issues such as heart disease, diabetes, depression, anxiety, and premature death. However, incorporating light physical activities into your daily routine can help combat the effects of a sedentary lifestyle. You don't need to spend hours at the gym; simply dedicating a short time each day to light exercise can significantly improve your health and protect against metabolic disorders.

The Role of Sleep in Mental Well-being

Many individuals are familiar with the notion that sleep significantly influences their mental well-being. It's commonly expressed through sayings like "waking up on the wrong side of the bed," reflecting the intuitive understanding that sleep quality can affect mood.

This familiar expression holds considerable truth. Sleep plays a vital role in mental and emotional health, with established connections to conditions such as depression, anxiety, bipolar disorder, and others.

Ongoing research aims to unravel the intricate, bidirectional relationship between mental health and sleep. While both are complex phenomena influenced by numerous factors, their close interconnection suggests that enhancing sleep quality could yield positive effects on mental well-being and may form part of the treatment approach for various psychiatric disorders.

How Does Sleep Impact Mental Health?
Sleep plays a crucial role in regulating brain activity, which fluctuates across different stages of the sleep cycle. These stages contribute to brain health by modulating activity levels

in various brain regions, thereby enhancing cognitive functions such as thinking, learning, and memory. Recent research has illuminated the profound influence of sleep-related brain activity on emotional and mental well-being.

Adequate sleep, particularly during rapid eye movement (REM) sleep, supports the brain's processing of emotional information. While asleep, the brain processes and consolidates thoughts and memories, with REM sleep being particularly instrumental in this regard. Conversely, insufficient sleep, especially the lack of REM sleep, can impede the consolidation of positive emotional content, thereby affecting mood, emotional responsiveness, and exacerbating mental health disorders. This association extends to an increased risk of suicidal ideation or behaviors. Consequently, the conventional view that regarded sleep problems solely as symptoms of mental health disorders is being reevaluated. Instead, emerging evidence suggests a bidirectional relationship between sleep and mental health, where sleep disturbances can both contribute to and result from mental health issues. Further exploration is warranted to delineate the intricate connections between sleep and mental health, including the myriad factors influencing this complex relationship on an individual level.

Additionally, obstructive sleep apnea (OSA) represents another facet of sleep that intersects with mental health. OSA, characterized by breathing pauses and decreased oxygen levels during sleep, disrupts sleep patterns and may exacerbate mental distress. Individuals with psychiatric conditions are more prone to OSA, heightening their vulnerability to physical health complications and worsening mental health outcomes.

The interconnectedness of sleep and mental health becomes increasingly evident when examining the relationship between sleep patterns and various specific mental health disorders and neurodevelopmental conditions.

Depression:

Depression affects over 300 million individuals globally, characterized by persistent feelings of sadness or hopelessness. Approximately 75% of those experiencing depression report symptoms of insomnia, alongside instances of excessive daytime sleepiness and hypersomnia, or oversleeping.

Traditionally, sleep disturbances were viewed as a consequence of depression. However, emerging evidence suggests that inadequate sleep may contribute to or worsen depressive symptoms. This bidirectional relationship suggests a reinforcing cycle where sleep problems and depression mutually impact each other.

While this cycle can perpetuate negative effects, it also presents an opportunity for innovative treatment approaches. Improving sleep quality may potentially alleviate symptoms of depression for some individuals, offering a promising avenue for holistic intervention.

Seasonal Affective Disorder (SAD):

Seasonal affective disorder is a form of depression that typically emerges during periods of decreased daylight, commonly affecting individuals in regions with limited sunlight, such as those in northern climates during autumn and winter.

This condition is intricately linked to disturbances in the body's internal biological clock, known as the circadian rhythm, which regulates various physiological functions, including sleep. Consequently, individuals with seasonal affective disorder often experience disruptions in their sleep patterns, characterized by either excessive or insufficient sleep, or alterations in their sleep cycles.

Anxiety Disorders:

Each year, anxiety disorders affect approximately 20% of adults and 25% of teenagers in the United States, manifesting as excessive fear or worry that can significantly impact daily functioning and pose risks for various health conditions, including heart disease and diabetes. These disorders encompass a range of conditions such as general anxiety disorder, social anxiety disorder, panic disorder, specific phobias, obsessive-compulsive disorder (OCD), and post-traumatic stress disorder (PTSD).

Anxiety disorders often co-occur with sleeping difficulties. The heightened state of worry and fear associated with anxiety contributes to a state of hyper-arousal, characterized by racing thoughts, which is a primary contributor to insomnia. Sleep disturbances, in turn, can exacerbate anxiety, leading to anticipatory anxiety at bedtime and making it challenging to initiate sleep.

PTSD, in particular, is strongly linked to sleep disturbances. Individuals with PTSD frequently experience intrusive memories, nightmares, and hyper vigilance, all of which can disrupt sleep patterns. This is notably prevalent among veterans, with up to 90% of combat-related PTSD sufferers experiencing symptoms of insomnia.

Furthermore, research suggests a bidirectional relationship between poor sleep and anxiety. While anxiety can contribute to sleep difficulties, chronic insomnia may predispose individuals to the development of anxiety disorders. Thus, addressing sleep disturbances is crucial in managing anxiety-related symptoms and preventing the onset of anxiety disorders.

Bipolar Disorder:

Bipolar disorder is characterized by alternating episodes of extreme mood swings, ranging from elevated highs (mania) to depressive lows. The symptoms and experiences vary significantly depending on the type of episode, yet both manic and depressive phases can significantly disrupt daily functioning.

Individuals with bipolar disorder often experience notable changes in their sleep patterns corresponding to their emotional state. During manic episodes, they typically require less sleep, whereas depressive periods may lead to excessive sleeping.

Evidence suggests that sleep disturbances can precipitate or exacerbate manic and depressive episodes, underscoring the bidirectional relationship between bipolar disorder and sleep. Consequently, addressing insomnia through treatment interventions may mitigate the impact of bipolar disorder symptoms.

Schizophrenia:

Schizophrenia is a mental health condition marked by challenges in distinguishing reality from fantasy. Individuals diagnosed with schizophrenia often encounter difficulties with sleep, including insomnia and disruptions in their circadian rhythms. Moreover, medications prescribed for schizophrenia treatment may exacerbate sleep disturbances. The interplay between poor sleep and schizophrenia symptoms can intensify each other, suggesting potential advantages in stabilizing and restoring normal sleep patterns as part of comprehensive treatment approaches.

Autism Spectrum Disorder (ASD):

Autism Spectrum Disorder (ASD) encompasses a range of neurodevelopmental conditions characterized by challenges in communication and social interaction, typically identified during early childhood and often persisting into adulthood.

Individuals with ASD, particularly children and adolescents, exhibit a heightened prevalence of sleep issues, including insomnia and sleep-related breathing difficulties. These sleep disturbances tend to be more enduring in individuals with ASD compared to those without the condition, and they can exacerbate symptoms and diminish overall quality of life. Prioritizing the management of insomnia and related sleep disruptions is integral to comprehensive care for individuals with ASD, as it has the potential to alleviate excessive daytime sleepiness and mitigate other associated health and behavioral concerns.

Strategies for Enhancing Sleep and Mental Health:

The intricate relationship between sleep and mental well-being underscores the complexity of their interconnections within psychiatric disorders. However, it also highlights the potential for concurrent treatment of both issues, where interventions aimed at improving sleep can complement mental health management and even serve as a preventive measure.

Given the unique circumstances of each individual, the most effective approach to addressing mental health and sleep concerns varies from person to person. Given the significant impact of these conditions on overall well-being, seeking appropriate care is crucial, necessitating collaboration with qualified healthcare professionals.

Medical doctors or psychiatrists are equipped to evaluate the potential advantages and drawbacks of various treatment modalities and offer personalized care, even in cases involving multiple concurrent physical or mental health conditions.

Cognitive Behavioral Therapy (CBT):
   Cognitive Behavioral Therapy (CBT) is a form of psychotherapy, also known as talk therapy, designed to explore and reshape patterns of thinking. By addressing negative thought patterns, individuals can work towards re-framing their thinking in more positive and constructive ways. Many individuals find that guidance from a trained therapist in altering their cognitive patterns can significantly enhance both their sleep quality and mental well-being.

Various forms of CBT have been tailored to address specific mental health challenges such as depression, anxiety, and bipolar disorder. Moreover, Cognitive Behavioral Therapy for Insomnia (CBT-I) has demonstrated effectiveness in alleviating sleep disturbances. Extensive clinical trials have further demonstrated that CBT-I can yield improvements in overall emotional health and reduce symptoms associated with various mental health disorders, thereby enhancing emotional stability and reducing instances of psychotic episodes.

Enhance Sleep Patterns:
   Poor sleep hygiene often underlies sleeping difficulties. Elevating sleep hygiene involves adopting habits and creating an environment in the bedroom that promotes restful sleep, thereby reducing disturbances during the night.

Examples of fostering healthier sleep patterns encompass:

- Establishing a consistent bedtime and adhering to a regular sleep schedule
- Incorporating relaxation techniques into a nightly routine to unwind before bedtime
- Avoiding consumption of alcohol, tobacco, and caffeine in the evening
- Diminishing light exposure and refraining from electronic device use at least an hour before bedtime
- Engaging in regular physical activity and exposure to natural light during the daytime
- Optimizing mattress, pillow, and bedding comfort and support
- Minimizing disruptions from excessive light and noise in the sleep environment
- Determining the most effective routines and bedroom setup may require experimentation, but this process can yield significant benefits by facilitating quicker sleep onset and maintaining uninterrupted sleep throughout the night.

Implementing Dietary Changes

You can improve your eating habits by making simple changes, like opting for whole grains instead of refined ones and increasing your protein intake. Scientific research confirms that a diet abundant in fruits and vegetables offers various health advantages, such as lowering the risk of chronic diseases and boosting the immune system.

Revamping your entire diet can feel daunting, so it might be easier to begin with small steps, like incorporating more of your preferred fruits, rather than attempting a complete overhaul all at once. This section explores strategies for gradually enhancing the nutritional quality of your usual diet.

Adjusting the presentation and timing of your meals

Opt for smaller plates

Your choice of dinnerware can impact how much you eat. Using larger plates can make portions appear smaller, while smaller plates can make them seem larger.

A 2017 study found that eating from smaller plates was associated with increased feelings of fullness and decreased calorie intake among individuals with a moderate body weight. Additionally, if you're unaware that you're eating less than usual, you're less likely to compensate by eating more later. By using smaller plates, you can deceive your brain into perceiving a larger meal, reducing the likelihood of overeating.

Start with greens

A practical way to ensure you consume your greens is to have them as an appetizer. Eating them when you're most hungry can lead to finishing them all, potentially resulting in consuming fewer, and possibly less nutritious, components of the meal later. This practice may contribute to overall calorie reduction and even weight loss. Furthermore, consuming vegetables before a meal rich in carbohydrates can help regulate blood sugar levels by slowing the absorption of carbs into the bloodstream, benefiting both short- and long-term blood sugar control, especially in individuals with diabetes.

Serve dressings, dips, and condiments separately

Ordering a salad at a restaurant is a commendable choice, but not all salads are equally healthy. Some may be laden with high-calorie dressings, making them more caloric than other menu options. Requesting dressings on the side allows for better portion control and calorie management.

Slow down

The speed at which you eat influences your food intake and the likelihood of weight gain. Research suggests that fast eaters tend to consume more and have a higher BMI compared to slow eaters. Your appetite, food intake, and satiety are regulated by hormones, but it takes about 20 minutes for your brain to receive these signals. Eating more slowly allows your brain the time it needs to recognize fullness, potentially reducing calorie consumption and aiding weight loss. Moreover, eating slowly is associated with thorough chewing, which is linked to improved weight management. Simply slowing down your eating pace and chewing more can help curb your appetite and promote healthier eating habits.

Grocery Shopping, Meal Planning, and Fast Food

Make a shopping list and avoid shopping on an empty stomach
When heading to the grocery store, it's essential to plan ahead by creating a shopping list beforehand and ensuring you're not hungry while shopping.

Shopping without a list can lead to impulse purchases, and hunger may tempt you to add more unhealthy items to your cart. By planning ahead and sticking to your list, you'll not only buy healthier options but also save money.

Steer clear of "diet" foods
Products labeled as "diet" or "low-fat" can be misleading. Although they may have reduced fat content, they often compensate with added sugar or other ingredients, resulting in higher calorie content. Instead, opt for whole foods like fruits and vegetables.

Cook meals at home more frequently
Making home-cooked meals a regular habit offers various

benefits. Firstly, it's usually more budget-friendly. Secondly, by preparing your meals, you have full control over the ingredients, eliminating concerns about hidden additives. Additionally, cooking in bulk provides leftovers for subsequent meals, ensuring satisfying and nutritious options.

Experiment with new recipes weekly

Break the cycle of repetitive meal choices by incorporating at least one new recipe into your weekly routine. Trying different recipes adds variety to your diet and exposes you to new nutrients and flavors.

Choose baking or roasting over grilling or frying

The method of food preparation significantly impacts its health effects. While grilling, frying, and deep-frying are popular cooking methods, they can produce potentially harmful compounds linked to health issues like cancer and heart disease. Opt for healthier cooking techniques such as baking, broiling, or poaching to minimize the formation of these compounds and promote healthier eating.

Select nutritious options when eating out

Eating out doesn't have to mean sacrificing nutrition. Look for fast-food restaurants or fusion kitchens that offer healthier menu choices to ensure you're making nutritious selections even when dining away from home.

Enhancing Your Diet with Nutrient-Rich Foods

Boost your protein consumption

Protein is often hailed as a crucial nutrient due to its remarkable effects on hunger and satiety hormones, making it exceptionally filling compared to other macronutrients.

A 2018 study revealed that consuming a high-protein meal reduced levels of ghrelin, the hunger hormone, more effectively than a high-carb meal, particularly among individuals with obesity. Additionally, protein aids in preserving muscle mass and may slightly elevate daily calorie expenditure. It's also essential for preventing muscle loss during weight loss and aging.

If weight loss is your goal, strive to incorporate a protein source into each meal and snack to promote prolonged satiety, curb cravings, and reduce the likelihood of overeating.

Excellent sources of protein include:

- Dairy products
- Nuts
- Peanut butter
- Eggs
- Beans
- Lean meats

Incorporate Greek yogurt into your daily meals

Greek yogurt, known for its thicker and creamier texture

compared to regular yogurt, undergoes a straining process to remove excess whey, resulting in a product with higher fat and protein content.

Consuming a protein-rich food like Greek yogurt can enhance feelings of fullness, aiding in appetite management and potentially reducing overall food intake, especially for those aiming to manage their weight. Additionally, Greek yogurt contains fewer carbohydrates and less lactose than regular yogurt, making it suitable for individuals following low-carb diets or those with lactose intolerance.

Opt for plain, unflavored varieties to avoid added sugars and less nutritious additives commonly found in flavored yogurts.

Incorporate eggs into your breakfast routine
    When compared to other breakfast options with similar calorie content, eggs consistently emerge as a top choice.

Eggs are packed with high-quality protein and essential nutrients like choline, often lacking in typical diets. Consuming eggs in the morning promotes feelings of fullness, resulting in reduced calorie intake during subsequent meals, which can be beneficial for weight management goals.

For instance, a 2020 study involving 50 participants found that consuming an egg-based breakfast led to decreased hunger and lower calorie consumption throughout the day compared to a cereal-based breakfast.

Healthy Swaps and Substitutions to Consider

Exchange sugary drinks for sparkling water
Sugary beverages are packed with added sugar, contributing to various diseases like heart disease, obesity, and type 2 diabetes. Unlike nutrient-rich foods, these drinks fail to regulate appetite effectively.

To cut down on empty calories and excess sugar intake, consider replacing sugary beverages with sugar-free alternatives or opting for still or sparkling water.

Occasionally enjoy black coffee
Coffee is rich in antioxidants and linked to numerous health benefits, including reduced risks of type 2 diabetes, cognitive decline, and chronic liver disease. However, commercial coffee varieties often contain added sugars, syrups, and heavy creams, compromising its health benefits.

To preserve coffee's health perks, try drinking it black or adding minimal amounts of milk or cream instead of sugar.

Opt for whole fruits over fruit juices
Whole fruits boast fiber and essential nutrients, offering health benefits such as reduced risks of heart disease, type 2 diabetes, and cancer. Unlike fruit juices, which lack fiber and may contain added sugars, whole fruits digest slowly, preventing blood sugar spikes.

Choose whole-grain bread over refined
Whole grains provide various health benefits, including

reduced risks of type 2 diabetes, heart disease, and cancer. Opt for bread made solely from whole grains, rich in fiber, B vitamins, zinc, and other essential nutrients.

Select popcorn over chips

Popcorn, a whole grain packed with nutrients and fiber, makes a nutritious snack compared to potato chips. Air-popped popcorn contains fewer calories and more fiber than potato chips, promoting satiety and reducing inflammation.

Enjoy fresh berries instead of dried ones

Berries are nutrient-dense and rich in antioxidants. Fresh berries offer a juicy, low-sugar snack compared to dried varieties, which are calorie-dense and often coated with added sugars.

Choose heart-healthy oils

Swap highly processed seed and vegetable oils for less processed options like extra virgin olive oil, avocado oil, or coconut oil. High omega-6 to omega-3 ratios in processed oils can lead to inflammation and increase the risk of chronic conditions.

Opt for baked potatoes over french fries

Baked or boiled potatoes provide fewer calories and less harmful compounds than deep-fried french fries. Swapping fries for baked potatoes reduces calorie intake and limits exposure to unhealthy compounds like trans fats.

Water Consumption

Ensure Adequate Hydration

Maintaining proper hydration is crucial for overall health.

Numerous studies have demonstrated that adequate water intake can facilitate weight loss and support weight management. Additionally, it may slightly elevate daily calorie expenditure. Drinking water before meals has also been shown to reduce appetite and subsequent food intake.

The key is prioritizing water over other beverages, which can significantly reduce sugar and calorie consumption.

In Summary

Attempting to overhaul your diet or lifestyle all at once can be overwhelming. Instead, consider gradually implementing some of the aforementioned changes one or two at a time to enhance your diet progressively.

These tips can assist in managing portion sizes, increasing nutrient intake, and adapting to new habits. Collectively, these adjustments can make a substantial difference in your overall health and well-being.

Overcoming Challenges and Barriers

One of these five factors might be hindering your progress towards reaching your nutritional objectives. Our dietitian offers advice to assist you in overcoming these obstacles to transformation. Altering your dietary habits can be difficult. Despite your sincere intentions, transitioning from unhealthy eating habits to a nutritious diet can pose challenges. If you find yourself grappling with improving your diet, you could be contending with one of the following prevalent obstacles. Our Wellness Dietitian, Lindsey Wohlford, provides suggestions to propel you forward if you encounter any of these impediments to change.

Time Constraints

Similar to any other goal you aim to accomplish, prioritizing healthy eating requires planning. Schedule dedicated time on your calendar for meal planning, grocery shopping, and meal preparation to ensure you have access to nutritious options.

Utilize time-saving strategies such as purchasing pre-cut fruits and vegetables, utilizing a slow-cooker, or doubling recipes to have leftovers for freezing. Maintain a list of quick, healthy meal and snack ideas to avoid feeling overwhelmed during shopping and cooking. Additionally, consider the convenience of online grocery shopping to streamline the process and save time.

Feeling Overwhelmed

Avoid attempting too many changes simultaneously. Incremental adjustments over time can yield significant results and are more manageable. Implementing drastic changes all at once can be daunting and challenging to sustain, leading to feelings of uncertainty.

By gradually mastering small changes, you'll build confidence, and these improvements will gradually integrate into your lifestyle. Once you've adopted a new habit, move on to the next one. Remember, change is a process, not an instant transformation.

An "All or Nothing" Mentality

Upon committing to change your eating habits, you might believe there's no room for errors. Eventually, setbacks and relapses are inevitable. Approaching change with an all-or-nothing mindset can turn setbacks into perceived failures, potentially causing you to give up.

Remind yourself that your goal is progress, not perfection. Treat setbacks as temporary obstacles and continue moving forward. Change requires time and persistence, but you'll reach your goals if you persevere.

Dietary Confusion

The abundance of trendy diets and various sources of nutrition information can create challenges and uncertainties when making healthy eating choices. This often results in experimenting with multiple diets and following nutrition advice lacking scientific evidence.

Consulting with a registered dietitian can help navigate through the misinformation and provide tailored, well-researched nutrition guidance that suits your individual needs and lifestyle. Dietitians also offer ongoing support, accountability, and encouragement.

Feeling Deprived

Embarking on a healthy lifestyle may involve giving up certain foods you enjoy. However, adopting a healthier diet does not necessarily require bidding farewell to all your favorites. All foods can be included in moderation, as a healthy diet emphasizes diversity and balance.

A dietitian can assist in understanding how to incorporate the foods you love while balancing them with other nutritious options to support weight management and reduce the risk of chronic diseases.

Identifying and addressing obstacles is essential for increasing the likelihood of success in achieving your health goals.

Meal Plan, with Exercises and Meditation

During challenging weeks when you need a mood or concentration boost, you can rely on this three-day meal plan and my personal tips to help restore your vitality and happiness. This approach has proven effective for me.

Maintain regular meal times to stabilize your blood sugar levels and safeguard your well-being. Avoid risking your happiness by skipping meals. On tough days, I ensure I have my favorite fruits readily available for snacks to prevent hunger from taking over.

Embrace the concept of "food as medicine" to support your mental health. For me, cooking serves as a therapeutic practice, allowing me to express creativity and find solace. Prioritizing nutritious meals positively impacts my overall well-being.

Recognize the importance of exercise as a vital component in managing mood disorders. Once I acknowledged its significance in maintaining emotional balance, I became more motivated and consistent in my exercise routine. Now, I understand that daily exercise is crucial for preventing anxiety.

During moments of heightened anxiety, I remind myself of the necessity to prioritize physical activity.

I ensure to engage in activities I genuinely enjoy, such as taking leisurely walks while listening to audio books or swimming in the ocean. Consistency is key, so adhering to a regular exercise schedule ensures I receive my daily "dose" of exercise therapy, effectively staving off anxiety symptoms.

Below is a three-day meal guide designed to enhance mental well-being and focus:

Day 1

Breakfast: Sun-drenched mushrooms served on sourdough with avocado

Exposing mushrooms to sunlight, even for a brief period, provides you with 100% of your daily Vitamin D requirement, a crucial nutrient for mood regulation.

Snack: Fresh fruit

Opt for a fruit variety you don't typically consume. Studies indicate that novelty can contribute to mood improvement.

Lunch: Fresh spinach salad paired with oven-roasted pumpkin, feta cheese, and pumpkin seeds

This combination of antioxidant-packed spinach, slow-releasing carbohydrates from pumpkin, and an abundance of healthy fats from feta cheese and seeds contributes to mood stabilization throughout the day.

Snack: A serving of Greek yogurt

Greek yogurt is rich in probiotics, which promote a healthy gut environment, known to correlate with improved mood. I personally incorporate a serving of probiotics into my daily routine.

Dinner: Enjoy a grilled salmon bowl accompanied by avocado, chickpeas, and a side of seasonal salad

Salmon is rich in both EPA and DHA, omega-3 fatty acids known for their positive effects on mood and concentration. Personally, I prefer Huon Salmon for its quality.

Exercise: Engage in a light jog. Incorporate 10 sprints uphill during your jog, followed by a leisurely walk downhill. This high-intensity interval workout stimulates the release of endorphins, boosting your mood. If you prefer a less intense workout, take a long walk with a pet or immerse yourself in an uplifting or inspiring podcast or book.

Mindfulness: Before retiring for the night, reflect on at least three things you're grateful for. Whether you jot them down or share them with your partner, make it a daily practice to cultivate gratitude.

Day 2

Breakfast: Indulge in sourdough toast topped with mashed avocado and a poached egg

Avocado and eggs are excellent sources of beneficial fats crucial for promoting a happier brain. I favor sourdough bread for its slower digestion, which helps maintain stable mood levels.

Snack: Enjoy a piece of fresh fruit

Opt for a different fruit variety compared to the previous day. Incorporating variety ensures a diverse intake of antioxidants, which are essential for nourishing a healthier mind.

Lunch: Enjoy a nourishing freekeh salad topped with walnuts

Freekeh, a flavorful whole grain, provides sustained energy, helping to maintain stable mood levels throughout the afternoon.

Snack: Treat yourself to Greek yogurt paired with frozen berries

Frozen berries offer a convenient and budget-friendly option rich in antioxidants, maintaining their nutritional value while providing a refreshing snack.

Dinner: Indulge in a zucchini noodle Pad Thai

Nourish your body with vegetables to support a healthier gut and uplifted mood. Incorporate nuts for a boost of healthy fats and protein.

Exercise: Attend a yoga class and immerse yourself in the present moment throughout the session. If your mind wanders to concerns, gently redirect your focus. Remind yourself of the importance of self-care and honoring your body. Investing in your well-being is always worthwhile.

Mindfulness: If you struggle with sleep, consider trying a guided gratitude meditation. Numerous free resources are available online. This practice can help you feel grounded and release worries, promoting restful sleep.

Day 3

Breakfast: Enjoy untoasted muesli served with natural yogurt and fresh fruit

Opt for slow-burning oats, probiotics-packed yogurt, and a variety of colorful fruits, providing a nourishing blend of nutrients and antioxidants.

Snack: Treat yourself to two peanut butter-stuffed dates

Savor this delightful sweet snack, rich in healthy fats, protein, and fiber from peanut butter, offering sustained energy and a mood boost.

Lunch: Indulge in a beef salad sandwich

Ensure you include enough iron in your diet, which is essential for maintaining energy levels, particularly found in beef.

Snack: Enjoy your preferred indulgence

I no longer completely eliminate my favorite treats from my diet. Instead, I allow myself to enjoy them mindfully once or twice a week.

Dinner: Delight in sweet potato boats filled with goat cheese and vegetables

Opt for lower glycemic index foods like sweet potato to maintain stable blood sugar levels and consequently, a balanced mood.

Exercise: Extend an invitation to a friend for a leisurely walk together. The social interaction will foster a sense of connection, while the physical activity will elevate your mood.

Mindfulness: Enhance your cooking experience by playing music while preparing dinner. This will allow you to savor the process and divert your attention from life stressors. When dining, make it a habit to sit at a table without distractions from a TV or phone, enabling you to fully enjoy your meals.

Conclusion

"Change Your Diet For Optimal Mental Health" empowers you to take charge of your well-being by harnessing the transformative power of nutrition. By understanding the profound impact of food on mental health, you hold the key to unlocking a brighter, more resilient mindset. Through simple dietary adjustments and mindful eating practices, you can pave the way towards a healthier, happier life. Remember, your journey towards optimal mental health begins with the choices you make at the dinner table. So, embrace this opportunity to nourish your body, uplift your spirit, and embark on a path towards lasting vitality.

Thanks

Thank you for journeying through "Change Your Diet For Optimal Mental Health." Your commitment to enhancing your well-being through nutrition is truly commendable. If you found value in the insights shared within these pages, I kindly invite you to leave a review and share your experience with others. Your feedback not only helps others discover the book but also strengthens our collective effort towards fostering mental wellness. Together, let's inspire and support each other on the path to optimal health.